How to Cheat Colds and Flu

A *FREE* DVD will be <u>posted</u> to purchases of this book. Simply forward your e-mail request to:
lifebuoy102@aol.com
Not forgetting your name and address!

Many people take it regularly for general health maintenance, finding that it strengthens their immune system, decreasing the incidence of colds and bronchial infections and flu.

Please see **Authors note** to claim your Free DVD.

NOTES

NOTES

How to Cheat Colds and Flu

Natural Healing and Remedies from the Hive

By Colin Platt

A GIFT FROM NATURE

How to Cheat Colds and Flu

Copyright © 2009 by Colin Platt

Disclaimer:
Every effort has been made to make this information as complete and accurate as possible up to the publication date. The author and webmaster do not warrant that the information in this eBook is fully complete and should be used as a guide only and no responsibility accepted for any errors or omissions.
The author and webmaster shall have neither liability nor responsibility to any person or entity with respect to any loss or damage caused or alleged to be caused directly or indirectly by this information. Additionally, see authors note on page 13.

Live your Life without Colds and Flu

"If you've ever experienced the agony of flu symptoms, a distressing cold or a chronic cough, when you feel that your lungs are on fire, you'll know that it can be a terrifying experience as you struggle to breathe".

"Now there is a safe natural way to combat these agonising symptoms, an antiviral product, lost for centuries. A powerful natural antibiotic to assist your own body's healing power naturally and boost your immune system."

Dear Colds and Flu Sufferer,

               "How to Cheat Colds and Flu" is a brand new eBook that you need to read and keep with you if you care about your health.

Like you, I accepted Colds and Flu as normal, often three or four bouts a year, sometimes with serious consequences, but *NOW YOU DON'T HAVE TO*.

As you study every word of this book you will be amazed at what you'll learn.

YOU CAN PUT IT TO WORK FOR YOU

RIGHT NOW because you'll be shown quickly and easily how to live without the misery of regular or annual attacks of colds and flu. Whilst others are badly suffering, you can sail through life with the minimum of discomfort.

"Prevention is better than cure"...this vital information is available to you immediately...

How do I know it works? Because I had bouts of colds and flu year after year with monotonous regularity until finally I had a chest infection so bad that I finished up in hospital on a ventilator unable to breathe, all caused by the onset of a common cold.

I've experienced how the effects of a cold and flu in particular can turn into life threatening events, and no way did I wish to experience another traumatic episode.

It became my mission, an obsession if you like, to never suffer again from colds and flu and then to do all I could to help others to overcome this common problem.

Over many months of diligent research I found many herbal remedies which seemed to ease the common cold symptoms, such as Garlic, Ginger, Echinacea vitamin C but I needed something which would **prevent** colds and flu.

I FOUND IT

It's been under our noses for centuries, but only available to the fortunate few.
Now it's your turn to learn about the amazing results this miracle natural product can bring to you.

My research ended with success 19 months later in 2008. The remedy had been there all the time under my nose! I found that it helped other medical problems and diseases too, much more about that later. I found that it.......

➢ Strengthened the immune system.

➢ A protection against the flu virus.

➢ Prevented re-occurring respiratory problems.

➢ Is an effective remedy to combat bronchitis

➢ It was used effectivelyover2000 years ago by the Ancient EGYPTIANS.

➢ Is a natural antibiotic alternative.

➢ Is a powerful natural antibacterial agent.

➢ Could help treat other illnesses.

COLD AND FLU FREE FOR THE PAST 7 YEARS

> *I was fortunate to discover this little known product more than 7 years ago, and I have no hesitation in recommending using this natural preventative remedy.*
>
> *C. Davis. York. UK*

Hippocrates (460-337 BC) reputed to be the 'father' of modern medicine recognised its antibacterial properties.

This eternal natural healer has been proven to not only to suppress colds and flu but to alleviate Sinus infections.

In the field of nutritional medicine our first line of defence is **prevention rather than cure.** Instead of waiting for infections to start and then using drugs from the pharmacy to kill the infectious bacteria we should adopt the ancient Chinese methods and strive to keep well rather than the reverse.

Fact... Even today in the USA the common cold leads to 75 to 100 million Physician visits per annum at a conservative cost of $7.5 billion, and in over the counter drugs Americans spend $2.9 billion and another $400 million on prescriptions for symptom relief. It's also a fact that the true cost to Industry and Commerce in terms of lost workdays, production costs and profits is almost incalculable, plus the personal cost in lost income and social activity.

 Now for a few cents per day you can save on these expensive Physician's visits and over the counter cures.

More than one third of patients who saw a doctor received an antibiotic prescription which adds up to 41 million prescriptions in the USA alone according to the world health organisation at a cost of $1 billion annually this of course has a massive implication for antibiotic resistance.

6

This constant overuse has contributed to mutations of bacteria into resistant strains turning simple infections into serious life threatening illnesses, over which we have less and less control. Doctor George Jacoby of the Harvard Medical School does not beat about the bush when he states that "Bugs are always figuring a way round the antibiotics we throw at them then they come roaring back." It would appear that bugs and bacteria are cleverer than man.

For a fraction of the cost I had found a remedy which didn't need antibiotics.

Here is a sample of what you will learn inside "How to Cheat Colds and Flu"

- ➢ How to say goodbye to harmful antibiotics.

- ➢ Fight your colds and flu the right way.

- ➢ Save upwards of $997 a year on medical bills.

- ➢ How to treat your children safely too.

- ➢ Alleviates throat infections

- ➢ Relieves halitosis (bad breath) and gum disorders

Transmission.

The common cold and flu is transmitted between people by one of two ways.

- In aerosol (sneezing) spray. Breathing it in.
- The entry point is through the nose and throat or from contaminated surfaces.

Flu or Influenza....Beat it for good.

Although often confused with the common cold, Flu is a more severe condition, causing a fever muscle pains a sore throat and coughing.... Think about it, **never having to seriously suffer** again from one of these agonising symptoms for days on end or even longer. But according to the World Health Organisation, tens of millions of people get flu which can be fatal, some, mostly the elderly and very young, die. Even healthy people can be affected at any age particularly those over 50 also very young children, who have chronic medical conditions, are more likely to get complications such as pneumonia sinus bronchitis and painful ear infections, so why take chances with yours and your family's health **When you don't have to.**

It's good to know need to know what you are up against, so, a brief explanation of the type 'A' virus which causes the most severe illness is interesting. It can be subdivided into different types.

- H1N1. Caused Spanish flu in 1918/1920 truly a global pandemic spreading even to the Arctic killing 40 to 100 million. 99% of deaths occurring in people under 65 and more than half in young adults in the 20 to 40 years age bracket old. This pandemic has been described as "THE greatest medical holocaust in history and may have killed as many people as the Black Death". **Swine Flu falls into this category.** Could this be the next Pandemic? This type of flu can be passed from person to person, simply by human contact, or contaminated surfaces, such as door handles, elevator buttons and public places.

- H2N2 Known as ASIAN Flu 1957-1958 killed 1 to 1.5 million.

- H3N2 Known as HONG KONG Flu killed .75 to 1 million.

- H5N1 or AVIAN FLU or bird flu as it is known, is the latest Pandemic threat 2008-2009 Due now, and known as the **"Coming Plague"** it is being taken very seriously indeed by responsible Governments particularly by the USA, UK and

Europe.   Flu jabs are being stockpiled in their million in anticipation of the immediate threat, but production is limited. Demand will exceed supply massively. So who will be selected, who will be prioritised?

The last place you want to go in the event of a pandemic is Hospital. They will be totally unprepared in a major event.

But we can help ourselves. Those with the knowledge of the natural preventative have proved its effectiveness time and time again. You will learn about it in "How to Cheat Colds and Flu".

Protection and prevention is in our hands **now**. It is **your** responsibility to protect yourself and keep healthy as no one else will.......

So You Have Two Choices

Be pro-active to yourself and your family and discover *How to Cheat Colds and Flu* and keep **these** dangerous ailments at bay with this proven natural sunshine remedy. The truth is, you cannot afford to take any more risks with your health, especially with increasingly resistant cold and flu strains on the horizon.

OR

Continue to be plagued by all these illnesses, and expensive physician's bills. Don't forget already the spectre of a 'superbug' (H5N1 Avian Flu) resistant to all known antibiotics is currently approaching, and it will be the **'Survival of the Fittest'**.

TABLE OF CONTENTS

INTRODUCTION

Congratulations! You've become one of many who are taking steps to protect themselves from the yearly onslaught of debilitating colds and flu and other common complaints and ailments.

Like you, I was tired of spending year after year on the miserable merry-go-round of contagious illness, battling the coughs, congestion, sore throats, sinus infections, body aches and fatigue of colds and flu. And like you, I didn't know there was a way to prevent these bouts of illness. I tried vitamin C, garlic, Echinacea and other herbs, which seemed to ease the symptoms, but didn't prevent me from getting sick in the first place.

I was on a quest to find something that would PREVENT me from contracting contagious illnesses, something that would strengthen my immune system and increase my natural defenses. I searched until I found it. Since then, I haven't had a cold, flu, or any other contagious illness. Now I want to pass that miracle remedy on to you.

Many people can't believe there's one miracle substance found in nature that possesses the key to fighting infection. This substance not only kills pathogens, but strengthens the body's immune system. Research has found the only substance in the world that's been proven to be antibiotic, anti-bacterial, anti-fungal AND anti-viral at the same time. An amazing by product of the bees that's been used for over 3,000 years and has also been proven through modern scientific research to do all of the above.

This miracle substance is Propolis. In reading this eBook, you'll learn everything you need to know about propolis, from its creation by bees, to its use by ancient Egyptians and Greeks, to the ways it can prevent and treat a myriad of illnesses.

You will also learn about the new super-bugs that have learned to outsmart antibiotics, but have been scientifically proven to be vanquished by propolis.

Some people think the chances of a natural substance like propolis successfully fighting antibiotic-resistant bacteria and killer viruses is about as likely as a **pet donkey winning the Kentucky Derby! Read on and you, like me, will have a new understanding of this miracle substance from the hive.**

I have not written this book for the sole purpose of converting you from using orthodox allopathic medicine, but to open your eyes to a natural product, that, although not in it's infancy, (as you will see as you read on), is a substance that you may know little about and which could be truly a benefit to you in it's use.

(Rather than ignore the catastrophic decline of our bee population I have added a brief comment on page 59 to the fact that we should all be aware of our bee predicament, and that we all have to contribute in keeping our environment clean and free of pesticides and manmade pollution.)

May this information bring you health, happiness, healing and miracles.

Nature and Science Reunited.

AUTHOR'S NOTE

Although every care has been taken to ensure that the information and material in this ebook on the uses of propolis and treatment of various ailments is accurate, it is not intended to be a guide to self diagnosis, self treatment and a substitute for a health care provider's consultation. The research is based upon personal experience by the author and others.
Never disregard expert medical advice or delay in seeking medical advice or attention due to the information contained in this publication.

The webmaster and author shall have neither liability nor responsibility to any person or entity with respect to any loss, damage, or injury directly or indirectly by the information contained in this book.

We must stress that where health is concerned, there is no substitute for seeking advice from a qualified physician or herbal practitioner, and should the reader have any questions on any articles contained herein, then the author and publisher strongly advise consulting a professional healthcare advisor.
If you have an allergic response to honey, bee stings, pollen, or Royal Jelly then medical advice is essential prior to the use of propolis.

Pregnant Women:

At the time of writing, clinical trials with propolis on pregnant women have not been evaluated so it would be wise to avoid using propolis at this time.
Avoid if you are breastfeeding.

Bee Stings:

If you are allergic to bee stings, then propolis could induce a side effect similar to a sting, inflammation, and redness of the skin.

Science and Nature Reunited.

CHAPTER 1

PROPOLIS: THE DEFENDER OF THE HIVE

Everybody knows that bees make honey, but few know the crucial part that propolis plays in the life cycle of the Western Honeybee (Apis mellifera). **The fact is, without propolis, there would be no bees, no hives and no honey.... FACT.**

What is propolis? Propolis (also called bee glue or bee putty) is a mixture of tree resin and bee secretions used in the construction and maintenance of beehives. Just like bees gather pollen and nectar to bring back to the hive for food, they collect plant resins to make propolis.

In Northern regions, the resins come primarily from poplar, pine and balsam trees. In southern climes, bees gather resins from certain flowers, as well as trees. After mixing it with a combination of saliva and beeswax, they stash the mixture in their storage sacs for the journey back to the hive.

Chemical analysis reveals that propolis is a complex amalgam of plant resin, beeswax, aromatic oils and bee pollen. Its hue varies from golden brown to almost black, with occasional green or red tints. Naturally, the color and the exact makeup of propolis varies according to the botanical source of the resin and the area of the bee's habitat.

It's no wonder the adage "Busy as a bee" was coined. Honeybees have been known to travel up to 12 square miles on pollen and resin gathering missions.

15

Propolis is to bees what penicillin is to various forms of bacteria, or at least, what penicillin *was* before bacteria learned to outsmart it. But the difference is, we don't encase our homes in penicillin to insure that they stay disease-free. Bees, those clever little engineers, *do* seal their homes with propolis to keep it sterile.

Because as many as 70,000 bees are apt to live in a single hive, it's imperative that the warm, dark, humid environment be kept free of mold, fungus and disease. And what bees have figured out in the 125 million years that they've been buzzing around earth, is that propolis is the most powerful antibacterial substance found in nature.

Bees use the sticky substance to line their walls and stop up cracks when they construct their hives. Virtually every surface in the hive is coated with a thin layer of the sterilizing substance. They also encase the hive entrance with a narrow tunnel of propolis. In order to get in and out of the hive, the bees must crawl through the tunnel, which cleanses them of dangerous bacteria and keeps the hive safe for its inhabitants. If by chance, a spider, or some other foreign body enters the hive that's too big to be carried out by the bees, they swath it in a thick cocoon of propolis, in effect mummifying it to ensure that it doesn't contaminate their home with mold or fungus.

Another clever use of propolis prevents one of bees' natural enemies from making a mass assault on their hive. Ants like honey (not to mention larvae and dead bees) as much, or more, than humans, and will go to great lengths to swarm into a hive en masse, kill the inhabitants and consume the delicious amber syrup within. Bees have devised an ingenious strategy to foil ant attacks using, you guessed it, propolis. Painting a thick layer of the sticky resin at the hive's entrance, the bees immobilize the ants long enough to sting them to death and thwart their attack.

Bees also spread a thin blanket of propolis over the cells of their honeycomb, keeping it bacteria free. This is crucial to the survival of the species, because honeycomb holds the hive's most important treasures (aside from the queen), bee larvae, pollen and honey.

Propolis also serves to reinforce the honeycomb, adding to its tensile strength. Perhaps this is why honeycomb, which is made primarily of wax, is able to hold loads of up to 25 times its weight in honey.

CHAPTER 2

A HISTORY OF PROPOLIS

It's believed that primitive humans enjoyed the fruits of the industrious little honeybee, dining on royal jelly, honey, honeycomb and larvae. However, it was the ancient Greeks who gave propolis the name we use today. *Pro*, means *before* and *polis*, refers to *city*. Thus, '*Before the city*' acknowledges that bees line the entrance of the hive with propolis, keeping it safe from infection and intruders. Some say that a more apt translation is, '*In defense of the city*'. And propolis truly is the defender of the city of bees, the hive.

About 3000 years before the Greeks used propolis; the Egyptians employed it in one of their most sacred rites, mummification. In order to preserve their dead and guarantee an auspicious afterlife, they melted down the whole beehive, honey, honeycomb, propolis, wax and all. Strips of linen were soaked in the mixture and wrapped around the body, forming an effective preservative cocoon to limit fungus, mold and decomposition.

The Greeks, as well as the Egyptians, Sumerians, Babylonians also immersed their dead in vats of honey, which served as a remarkably effective preservative. Alexander the Great is among several notable Greeks who received a honey immersion burial.

The philosopher and scholar Aristotle (around 350 BC) was the first to undertake detailed research on the antiseptic and healing properties of propolis. He built a glass hive to better observe honeybee workings, but the bees, preferring to conduct their business in darkness, promptly coated the glass in propolis. Despite the bees desire to obscure their nest, Aristotle gleaned significant insight into their realm and made noteworthy advances in the knowledge of their industry. He chronicled the antiseptic quality of propolis and recommended its use for a variety of ailments, including bruises and sprains.

Hippocrates, holder of the illustrious title, "father of modern medicine", prescribed propolis for sores and ulcers. The Greeks were the first known civilization to promote beekeeping as an endeavor worthy of cultivation. The healthful properties of bee products became so well known throughout Greece, that they boasted as many as 20,000 cultivated hives by the year 400 BC.

Propolis was the primary ingredient of prized incense used in ancient Greece. Mixed with aromatic herbs and burned on charcoal, it emitted a delicate, but sublime perfume.

In Rome, Pliny the Elder (23 – 79 AD) further advanced the knowledge of propolis in his treatise *Natural History*, identifying three distinct types of the substance. He noted that propolis was commonly prescribed by physicians to reduce swelling, extract material embedded in the flesh, and heal wounds that were so severe as to have been deemed incurable.

References have been found in the Koran to the medicinal properties of honey and propolis, confirming that the ancient Arabic world was also in tune with apiarian remedies.

Eastern European medical journals from the 13th century document the use of propolis to relieve tooth decay. It's also known to have been used as a remedy for inflammations, abscesses, canker sores and respiratory infections. Because of its anti-bacterial and anti-fungal properties, propolis was used to treat wounds during the Boer Wars in South Africa in the late 1800's. It was dubbed 'Russian Penicillin' in World War II, when the Soviet military used it as wound dressing.

A piece of propolis slowly dissolved in the mouth is an age old sore throat and canker sore remedy recommended by beekeepers. Propolis lozenges are sold all over the world to heal and soothe a sore throat.

Although bee-product remedies were largely discarded in the West in favor of synthetic pharmaceuticals in the latter part of the 20th Century, their resurgence is burgeoning, particularly as modern antibiotics are proving increasingly ineffective against mutating strains of viruses and bacteria.

Healthcare providers are seeking new ways of staving off potentially catastrophic epidemics which modern pharmaceuticals are unable to treat. Could it be that a centuries-old product from the hive will reemerge as the magic bullet they've been looking for?

World-renowned Stradivarius violins were crafted in Italy in the late-1600's-early-1700. Antonio Stradivari used propolis in his varnishes, which is believed to have enhanced their beauty and clarity of tone.

Chapter 3

Super-Bugs, a Worldwide Threat

Today's headlines are full of alarming news about so-called 'super-bugs' that are immune to modern pharmaceutical treatment. Epidemiologists are increasingly concerned about these new, rapidly mutating viruses and antibiotic-resistant bacteria with the potential to infect billions of people. The potential for a world wide pandemic is enormous.

A review of some of the findings:

➤ In the United States, the Journal of the American Medical Association reported that over 94,000 people were infected with antibiotic-resistant staphylococcus in 2005. Of those 94,000 people, 18,650, or roughly 20 percent, died of the infection.

➤ In Europe, studies show that resistant streptococcus pneumonia has become resistant to penicillin almost 50 percent of the time. Other reports reveal that large numbers of soldiers returning from Afghanistan and Iraq have contracted wound infections that are resistant to antibiotics.

➤ Flesh-eating bacteria (necrotizing fasciitis) are also cause for concern. A little over a year ago, a woman in the U.S. had almost half of her upper body (hand, arm, shoulder and breast) sequentially amputated after she was attacked by the infection, which is caused by an antibiotic-resistant form of strep A. She was fortunate - the disease usually kills its victims within 72 hours.

➢ Avian or bird flu is first known to have morphed from chickens to humans in 1997. Because of its resistance to all known antiviral medications, experts believe the H5N1 virus has the ability to become a worldwide pandemic, killing billions of people. It had a 50 percent mortality rate when it spread throughout Asia in 2003 and has since cropped up in Africa, Europe and the Middle East, causing the deaths of over 200 people and killing an estimated hundreds of millions of birds. Currently the virus is only known to have the ability to be passed from infected birds to humans, but epidemiologists fear that it may have discovered a way to be transmitted from human to human.(See more on this subject in Chapter 7.)

Twenty-five million pounds of antibiotics, or 70% of all the antibiotics produced are fed to livestock in the U.S. each year. Because of repeated exposure to antibiotics, pathogens have morphed into more resistant strains in order to survive.

➢ Although health experts thought that modern antibiotics had relegated tuberculosis to the dustbin of medical history, they've recently had cause to reconsider. A new, virtually untreatable form of tuberculosis (XDR-TB) is impervious to antibiotics. The strain has cropped up in India, causing alarmingly high mortality rates. The World Health Organization fears that XDR-TB is set to become a deadly global health threat.

These kinds outbreaks have prompted the U.S. Center For Disease Control to state that antibiotic-resistant bacteria is one of the world's most pressing problems, adding that, "Over the last decade, almost every type of bacteria has become stronger and less responsive to antibiotic treatment."

Researchers believe that the reason for this is twofold: First, the widespread overuse of antibiotics by the general public. Since penicillin was invented in the 1940s, people have learned to rely on antibiotics to an extreme degree. Doctors, often at the patient's insistence, will prescribe antibiotics at the drop of a hat, even for maladies like viral infections on which they have no remedial effect whatsoever.

Secondly, the use of antibiotics in livestock: Although the use of antibiotics as a preventative treatment in the commercial livestock industry has been largely banned throughout the EU, the U.S. still employs the practice, pumping huge quantities of the drugs into animal feed. In industrial style livestock production, antibiotics ameliorate the negative health effects of overcrowding and unsanitary conditions.

Bacteria have learned to survive on the earth longer than man or beast. In fact, bacteria are the first forms of life on earth and have been around for four billion years. Like all living things, they have their own innate intelligence and ability to evolve in a way that guarantees their survival.

Bees, it seems, have found a way to beat bacteria at the survival game with a miraculous substance created from plant resins. If we want to protect ourselves from constantly evolving pathogens, we can take a lesson from the bees and turn to propolis to safeguard our most important possession, our health.

> *Unlike antibiotics, we can take propolis daily as a preventative measure to strengthen our immunity to a vast array of illnesses.*

Chapter 4

**The Good News: A Miracle Antibiotic
From the Hive**

As you learned in earlier chapters, propolis possesses a phenomenal array of curative properties, including anti-fungal, antibacterial, anti-inflammatory, antibiotic, antacid and anti-tumor.

It's used to treat a wide spectrum of health problems: arthritis, muscle soreness, respiratory illness, skin disorders, wounds, chronic fatigue syndrome, burns, tooth decay, allergies, endometriosis, menstrual cramps, candida, infertility, prostate inflammation, urinary tract infections, ulcers, laryngitis, parasites, chronic fatigue syndrome, smallpox, herpes, canker sores, tumors and digestive disorders.

How many times have you come in contact with a fellow worker who thinks they're doing everyone a favor by coming to work with a cold or flu? This walking petri dish, sniffling, sneezing, coughing and generally infecting everyone around them, will no longer be cause for alarm if you're fortifying your defenses with propolis!

Many people now take it regularly for general health maintenance, finding that it strengthens their immune system, decreasing the incidence of colds and bronchial infections and flu.

With a fortified immune system, we can keep ourselves healthy in even the most virus and germ infected environments. There are many testimonials from people who used to get colds and flu every year. Since taking propolis, they've breezed through cold and flu season with nary a sneeze, ache, sore throat or sniffle. Medical researchers, for whom modern synthetic drugs were once a Holy Grail, have tried to determine why propolis is able to treat such a vast number of disorders.

They attempted to isolate the various chemical properties of propolis in hopes of finding one active component that's responsible for its effects. Because it has more than 150 chemical properties and because those chemical components depend on the botanical source, propolis is difficult to analyze. Nevertheless, researchers have found that no one component is responsible for curative effects of propolis.

In fact, when the chemical components of propolis are isolated, they don't work effectively. Rather, propolis combines all of its properties to create a synergistic effect.

Interestingly, propolis doesn't just destroy pathogens, it also boosts the body's immune system, allowing it to pull the trigger on disease without destructive side effects.

In simple terms, it's the sum of its parts, rather than any one component that enables this miracle from nature's pharmacy to do its curative work.

Another property of propolis is that, unlike synthetic antibiotics, it doesn't destroy the good bacteria with the bad. Anyone who's taken antibiotics and has come down with a yeast infection, an upset stomach, or diarrhea, knows that synthetic antibiotics are undiscriminating in their war on bacteria. Because our bodies maintain a complex system of bacterial equilibrium in order to stay healthy, destroying bacteria indiscriminately creates its own set of problems. This is another reason why propolis is so special.

We might use this analogy in describing propolis use: If our bodies were a castle in danger of being invaded by an army of enemy marauders, it would make more sense to reinforce the wall surrounding the castle, rather than to set off a bomb which would indiscriminately destroy the wall and the marauders alike.

Propolis is also shown to work in conjunction with synthetic antibiotics. Studies in Brazil, Australia and Bulgaria show that it boosts the efficacy of Penicillin and other antibiotics by as much as 100 percent.

Another study using propolis in conjunction with amoxicillin, ampicillin and cefalexin in fighting salmonella showed a synergistic effect in increasing efficacy. Propolis also reduces the amount of synthetic antibiotics administered to patients, thus reducing the side effects.

What are the chemical compounds of this miracle healer? Forty to fifty percent of propolis is made up of resins, which are rich in flavonoids.

Flavonoids exist in all blossoming plants, but they have different properties when found in propolis. Experts believe that the enzymes excreted in bee saliva when the bees process propolis produce a chemical change in the flavonoids.

> *Flavonoids comprise as much as 20 percent of the biochemical properties of propolis, which might explain why it's such powerful natural healing agent.*

There are many different types of flavonoids, but the most important ones found in propolis are pinocembrin and galangin, which have significant therapeutic properties. Flavonoids are shown to strengthen the protein shell surrounding viruses, which renders the virus harmless. It also stimulates the production of interferon, which stimulates the immune system.

Propolis has phenolic compounds, including caffeic acid phenethyl ester, which has been shown to inhibit the growth of cancer cells and reduce inflammation.

Propolis also contains essential minerals and trace elements such as calcium, magnesium, copper, potassium, manganese, phosphorus, iron, cobalt, silica and zinc. Perhaps most importantly, propolis can be taken regularly as a preventative, health-boosting measure, insuring good health and vitality and keeping illness at bay, no matter what the circumstance.

It's important to note that propolis may cause an allergic reaction in some people. You should take the necessary precautions when you begin using propolis, by taking only very small quantities at first. Once you determine that you don't have an allergy to it, you can begin taking a full dose. You are more likely to be allergic to propolis if:

❖ You have a severe allergy to bee stings.

❖ You are allergic to bee pollen or honey.

❖ You are allergic to evergreens, poplar or balsam trees.

❖ You have asthma.

You should also avoid using propolis if you are pregnant or nursing, just as you would take precaution when using any form of medication.

Do not stop using prescribed medication without consulting a professional medical practitioner.

To sum it up: propolis is one of the most powerful natural healing agents known to man. It has the ability to disarm a wide variety of pathogens and cure a vast array of illnesses.

Chapter 5

Scientific Studies on Propolis

As worldwide health organizations recognize that modern pharmaceuticals are becoming ineffective in combating illness-causing bacteria and viruses; they begin to look for alternative treatments. But the fact is, scientific research on the health effects of propolis has been going on for over forty years.

Western research on propolis began in the 1960's in Denmark and France with studies by Dr. Remy Chauvin and Dr. Aagard Lund. Dr. Chauvin, who conducts his research at the Sorbonne in Paris, is considered the world's foremost authority on propolis. Dr. Aagard developed a process of cleaning and preserving propolis that is still considered state-of-the-art today.

> *Chauvin also points out that propolis bestows significant amounts of vitamins and minerals when taken internally, while antibiotics do the opposite, causing deficiencies in these important nutrients.*

Chauvin states, "Scientists believe that nature has a cure for every disease. It's just a matter of finding it. With the introduction of propolis, it is possible that we can one day abolish most drug-related chemicals. Also, remember that keeping the body free from diseases through natural healing can actually slow down the aging process and add years to the lifespan."Chauvin says, "The antibacterial and antiviral properties of propolis work to raise the body's natural resistance to disease by internally stimulating one's own immune system. Since Chauvin began to tout the miracle healing powers of propolis, scientific studies on the subject have risen dramatically, with over 300 scientific studies conducted on propolis between 1980 and 2003, and the numbers increasing in the new millennium.

These studies verify what the ancients learned centuries ago: propolis is truly a miracle healer, capable of eradicating both viruses and bacterial infections, something no other substance is known to do.

Some of the recent research conducted on propolis:

❖ Researchers at the University of Western Australia have found that propolis can increase the effectiveness of penicillin or other antibiotics anywhere from 10 to 100 times. Studies done in Bulgaria and Brazil corroberate this finding.

❖ Research by Dr. Ali F. M. at the Ain Shams University in Egypt found that propolis successfully treats infertility associated with mild endometriosis with virtually no side effects.

❖ Research done at the Department of Microbiology, University of Alabama at Birmingham confirmed the existence of anti-microbial agents in various bee products, using streptococci bacteria as a test.

A study at the Instituto de Ciências Biomédicas da Universidade de São Paulo, Brazil and the Graduate Institute of Food Science and Technology at National Taiwan University, both concluded that propolis inhibits the growth of Staphylococcus aureus.

❖ The Department of Science at the Università degli Studi di Roma La Sapienza, Roma, Italy studied ethanolic extract of propolis (EEP) in conjunction with antibacterial drugs on Staphylococcus aureus. The scientists concluded: "Our results indicated that EEP had a significant anti-microbial activity towards all tested clinical strains."

Adding EEP to antibacterial tested drugs, it drastically increased the anti-microbial effect of ampicillin, gentamycin and streptomycin, moderately the one of chloramphenicol, ceftriaxon and vancomycin, while there was no effect with erithromycin. Moreover, our results pointed out an inhibitory action of EEP on lipase activity of 18 Staphylococcus spp. strains and an inhibitory effect on coagulase of 11 S. aureus tested strains."

❖ The Department of Microbiology and Immunology, Silesian Academy of Medicine, Zabrze-Rokitnica, Poland concluded: "Ethanolic extract of propolis exerts a strong anti-bacterial activity, in addition to anti-fungal, antiviral and anti-protozoal properties. In previous studies at these laboratories we have demonstrated that the intensity of the bactericidal activity of EEP is correlated with the virulence of the mycobacteria tested, and that EEP has a synergistic effect with antibiotics on growth of staphylococcus aureus."

❖ The Department of Biochemistry, University of Oxford, United Kingdom conducted research on: "The effect of the natural bee product propolis on the physiology of microorganisms was investigated using B. subtilis, E. coli and R. sphaeroides. An ethanolic extract of propolis had a bactericidal effect caused by the presence of very active, but labile, ingredients. The exact bactericidal effect of propolis was species dependent: it was effective against gram-positive and some gram-negative bacteria. Propolis and some of its cinnamic and flavonoid components were found to uncouple the energy transducing cytoplasmic membrane and to inhibit bacterial motility.

❖ The Departamento de Microbiologia, Laboratório de Biologia de Microrganismos in Brazil conducted a study of propolis ethanolic extract for inhibitory activity against periodontitis causing bacteria. Their results stated, "All of the assayed bacterium species were susceptible to propolis extract.

❖ The Department of Oral Biology, Faculty of Dentistry, Hebrew University-Hadassah, in Jerusalem, Israel conducted the following

29

study: "To investigate the antibacterial properties of propolis and honey against oral bacteria in vitro" (in an artificial environment) and in vivo (in a living organism.) RESULTS: Propolis demonstrated an Antibacterial effect both in vitro on isolated oral streptococci and in the clinical study on salivary bacterial counts.

CHAPTER 6

FORMS OF PROPOLIS

Because of increased awareness of the vast array of healing properties of propolis, it is now available in a variety of forms and can be purchased at most health food stores and many pharmacies.

Propolis preservation was first researched by Dr. Aagard Lund, mentioned in Chapter 5 for his propolis work in the 1960's and 1970's. Lund was the first to develop a process for preserving propolis. His process is still used by many producers today to insure the integrity of propolis's healing properties.

After propolis is gathered and cleaned of extraneous material, the active components are extracted by soaking it in alcohol. Then the mixture is dehydrated, either using a vacuum process, a spray process or a freezing process, at which time a wide variety of propolis products are produced, such as:

Just as you would with any product, it is important to get propolis from a reputable source. Because propolis is extremely sticky, it absorbs pollutants from the air. Therefore, it's important to get propolis that's been harvested in an area that's relatively orally for a variety of ailments.

- Capsules: These are available in two forms, either liquid propolis encased in capsules; or powdered propolis, encased in capsules. Both are taken

31

- Tinctures: Propolis in a base of water, alcohol or propylene glycol. Can be taken internally or externally, though it can stain the skin if applied externally.

- Lozenges: Propolis extract prepared with honey or sugar. Used for sore throats and coughs.

- Throat spray: Good sore throat soother.

- Nasal spray: Used for inflamed and clogged sinus passages. Both nasal and throat aerosols can be used for halitosis or mouth sores. Can also be used externally for cuts, rashes and fungal infections.

- Cough syrup: Soothes a sore throat and inflamed bronchial tissues, thus quieting a cough.

- Creams: Usually a 2% liquid propolis solution mixed in a cream base. Used for skin problems such as eczema, dermatitis, psoriasis and burns. Also used as an anti-aging cream because of its ability to improve skin elasticity.

- Ointments: Same preparation as with the cream, but the propolis is mixed in an oil base. Used for the same conditions as cream.

- Shampoo: Propolis extract added to shampoo formula. Used to invigorate and nourish the scalp and hair. Can stain hair, so it needs to be a low propolis concentration.

- Soap: Especially good for acne treatment and other skin conditions.

- Toothpaste: Good preventative for gum disease and halitosis.

- Gum: Believed to help dental hygiene and halitosis.

- Lip balm: Used to treat chapped lips and cold sores.

A list of conditions and treatment options with propolis:

> Acne: Propolis cream, ointment, capsule or tincture.

> Burns: Propolis cream, ointment, tincture, lip balm.

> Colds and coughs: Propolis capsule, tincture, cough syrup.

> Dermatitis: Propolis cream, ointment, tincture, lip balm.

> Eczema: Propolis cream, ointment, lip balm.

> Gum problems: Propolis capsule, tincture, toothpaste, chewing gum.

> Health Maintenance: Propolis capsule, tincture.

> Herpes: Propolis cream, ointment, tincture, lip balm.

> Laryngitis: Propolis capsule, tincture, cough syrup.

> Sore throat: Propolis capsule, tincture, cough syrup.

> Yeast infections: Propolis cream, capsule, ointment, tincture.

Despite the plethora of packaged propolis products, it's believed that the best way to administer it is to chew the pure form taken directly from the hive. Care should be exercised if taking scrapings from the floor of the hive as they might contain debris and impurities
.
The visible impurities are most likely to be small slivers of timber or wood from the hive, as the bees make sure that there is a good seal to cover any cracks and ingress of water.
If the beekeeper does not attend the hive regularly then the propolis can harden and more force has to be used with sometimes cosmetic damage to the hive.

Again, use propolis in tiny quantities until you determine that you don't have an allergy to it. The allergy can be in the form of itchiness of the skin, maybe a rash and skin irritation. Do not use if you have a bee allergy, or if you are pregnant or nursing.

Do not stop using prescribed medication without consulting a professional medical practitioner.

CHAPTER 7

A GLOBAL HEALTH CRISIS
IN THE MAKING: AVIAN FLU

Unfortunately, just because avian influenza (also known as bird flu, or H5N1 virus) has all but disappeared from the headlines, doesn't mean we can rest easy.

Avian flu is currently one of the deadliest viruses in the world, with the potential to kill billions of people. There is currently no known way of controlling the spread of avian flu. No one will be immune to it.

In March of 2008, the United Nations Food and Agriculture Organization (FAO) issued a warning that the risk of an avian flu mutation into a human pandemic form is growing increasingly dire.

The chief veterinary officer of the UN's FAO says that unless the disease is contained at its source in animals, there will be many more cases of transmission to humans. Currently the virus can only be passed from birds to humans, but the more human cases of H5N1, the more likely it is that the virus will learn how to mutate from human-to-human. Once it evolves into a form that can be transmitted within the human species, a worldwide epidemic of historic proportions will likely follow.

There are two methods by which H5N1 can improve its ability to be transmitted among humans. The first is what scientists call a 'reassortment event', whereby human and avian viruses exchange genetic material. This would occur during simultaneous infection of a human or a pig. In this case, the virus would obtain the ability to infect humans, exploding into a worldwide pandemic.

> *In Indonesia and Egypt, the virus appears to have mutated into a new strain, rendering attempts to develop a vaccine useless.*

The second method of evolution happens when the virus gradually develops the ability to bind to human cells. This involves small clusters of human avian influenza infections, with some incidence of human-to-human transmission. According to some accounts, this may already be occurring.

The first known human outbreak of avian influenza linked directly to chickens was in Hong Kong in 1997. Since then, the virus has spread throughout Asia, also making its route through Egypt, Turkey and Romania.

> *The virus can be transmitted by touching contaminated surfaces. Anyone who comes in contact with someone with the virus runs the risk of contracting it.*

Indonesia is the biggest source of avian influenza, with an estimated 30 million people continuing to raise chickens in close proximity to humans, despite the health risk. Indonesia has reported 129 cases of the virus to date. Of those known cases, 105, or 81 percent, were fatal.

H5N1 is highly contagious from poultry contact. Anyone working with poultry, eating undercooked poultry, or traveling in a country affected by the virus is at increased risk for contracting the avian flu. The movement of H5N1 virus into wild bird populations further increases the risk of an epidemic. A survey in the EU found 741 cases of avian flu in wild birds between February and May of 2006. The birds were identified in the UK, France, Greece, Italy, Hungary, Slovenia, Germany, Austria, Slovakia, Sweden, Poland,

Most of the infected wild birds have been swans, but ducks, geese and birds of prey have also found to carry the virus. The good news: propolis, with its ability to kill virus pathogens, may be the best bet when it comes to protecting ourselves against avian flu. At this point, no scientific studies have been done to determine propolis's effect on the H5N1 virus. However, it's quite possible that the most powerful anti-viral, anti-bacterial, anti-fungal substance found in nature will also prove effective in fighting avian flu.

No other substance has the ability to boost the immune system and eliminate pathogens. Propolis could very well divert a devastating avian influenza pandemic, which currently has no other means of remedy.

More H5N1 facts (from The World Health Organization):

- ❖ Domestic ducks now appear to be silent bearers of avian flu, having developed the ability to infect other birds without exhibiting symptoms of the illness. They excrete large amounts of the virus in their feces, further increasing the risk of spreading the disease. Because they do not appear to be sick, humans and other birds are more likely to come in contact with infected ducks, thus increasing transmission of the virus.

- ❖ Researchers have compared the H5N1viruses from 1997 and 2004, and found that they've become more deadly and are able to survive longer in the environment.

- ❖ Avian flu has widened its host range. It now infects and kills mammals that were previously considered resistant to infection with the virus. An unprecedented die-off of wild birds occurred in China in 2005, when more than 6,000 migratory birds were killed by avian flu.

- ❖ The 1918 flu pandemic killed an estimated 40 million people. An avian flu epidemic is expected to have a much higher mortality rate.

- ❖ Because of the large numbers of people requiring medical treatment, health services will be overwhelmed by an avian flu pandemic. High rates of health worker infection will further hamper attempts to treat the sick.

- ❖ Other essential services, such as transportation, communications, governmental and law enforcement agencies will be negatively impacted in their ability to function, due to worker infection.

❖ The ability of international relief organizations to offer assistance during a pandemic will likely be suspended, due to the need to contain the spread of the virus by limiting travel.

❖ Because the H5N1 virus is constantly mutating, vaccines are not expected to become available until several months after the start of an epidemic. Current vaccine production capacity falls far short of the amount needed to treat a pandemic.

❖ There are currently only two drugs known to treat influenza, oseltamivir (Tamiflu) and zanamivi (Relenza). Both must be administered within 48 hours of the onset of symptoms. There is no clinical proof that these drugs are effective against the H5N1 virus.

At current manufacturing capacity, it will take at least 10 years to produce enough of the above-mentioned drugs to treat just 20 percent of the world's population. The bottom line, propolis, the miracle remedy from the hive, could help stave off a killer flu pandemic in two ways: 1) It strengthens the immune system, enabling the body to use its own infection-fighting defenses more effectively and 2) by its ability to kill deadly pathogens, including viruses, on contact.

Avian flu or bird flu (H5N1) is a very serious threat. The World Health Organization (W.H.O.) fears that avian flu could kill millions in the next few years given the high volume of global traffic.

Chapter 8

Conditions Helped with Propolis

The Russians have probably done the most research in discovering the antibiotic, anti-inflammatory, and antibacterial properties of propolis in 1947 at the Kazan Veterinary Institute, so much so that propolis came to be known as 'Russian penicillin', prior to this date, it was being used and applied to slow healing wounds during the Boer War, and again during the Second World War in Russia.

Reports in the use of this amazing substance have become legendary. When Dr. Bernard Jenson Ph.D. visited the Caucasus people in Russia he found that, "All the oldest men in the area had been beekeepers and used raw honey AND hive scrapings as a regular part of their diet."He interviewed one of the beekeepers Shirali Mislimov who was 157 years old!

Colds and Coughs

In 1989 Polish researchers gauged the effects of propolis on groups with the common cold. The group treated with propolis had the infection for a shorter period, with complete recovery within 3 days. The untreated group took five days to recover. Research into it's uses showed that it is more effective as a **prophylactic** i.e. preventing catching the ailment rather than curing it. The old adage 'prevention is better than cure' rings true!
Self Help.........researchers find that the best results seem to be obtained by taking 1 to 1.5 grams per day, but do recommend backing off for a week every three months to prevent the body becoming over sensitized

Influenza (Flu)

We all know that flu is a viral infection and that as a rule antibiotics are not medically prescribed, as they are of little value, except in cases of a severe respiratory infection. I have found, and other propolis users have also confirmed that one is less likely to catch flu, but if you do suffer it is not as severe.

In May 1976 a particular virulent Flu epidemic swept through the town of Sarajevo.
Professor Izet Osmanagic a local resident conducted a trial and chose a control group who were in particular danger of becoming exposed to the epidemic, namely, student nurses and teachers.
Each was instructed to take propolis and honey every day for a certain period.
Sixty five nurses and teachers who were without symptoms took the product and 157 did not.
Only about one in ten of the students who took propolis were infected and out of the 157 in the control group, one in four contracted the epidemic.
The teachers faired even better as only one in twenty five had a mild attack.

Dr. Kravcuk of Kiev found that propolis was effective against sore throats and dry coughs in ninety percent out of two hundred and sixty cases.

Dr. Remy Chauvin of Paris, France concurs. "Propolis works by raising the body's natural resistance to infection; through stimulating ones own immune system.

Dosage to Help:
To stay well up to 2 grams daily, in capsule or tablet form.

Although I have researched and used propolis extensively, during my studies of the subject I have come across a wide range of benefits attributed to this amazing natural product, ranging from Acne to Ulcers!

Let me table for you, some of the wide ranging results, as confirmed by a world authority James Fearnley.

In James Fernley's book "Bee Propolis" 2001, he tables user's experiences with Propolis as follows:

	Positive	Negative	Too Soon
Arthritis and muscular pain:	89%	7%	4%
General health maintenance:	89%	0%	11%
Respiratory problems:	76%	7%	17%
Skin problems:	90%	9%	1%
Chronic fatigue syndrome:	63%	16%	21%
Stomach and digestive disorders:	69%	9%	22%

Acne and skin problems

It can be seen from the table above that skin problems scored a 90% positive result in the use of propolis. Many people have reported suffering with Acne for years, and applying propolis cream has shown its effectiveness within just a few weeks.
A tincture of propolis can be used but it can have a temporary staining effect on the skin.

Doctor Edith Lauder of Vienna in her clinic used propolis tinctures and creams on more than twenty cases of *acne simplex* which were completely healed by home application within a week.
Her most memorable result was in the treating of a woman who had been treated unsuccessfully for thirty years with *acne conglobata* on her face and chin. The condition was cleared after just a few visits to her clinic. She had many more notable successes in treating dermatology conditions.

Dosage to help:
Use Propolis cream and tinctures.(Tinctures can stain the skin). Propolis soap is now available, and. its use can be recommended for acne treatment.

Arthritis

The above table is a positive indication of the effectiveness of propolis.
Many people are unable to take anti-inflammatory medication due mainly to the adverse effect it has on the lining of the stomach, and have turned to this more natural product.
A poultice consisting of least 10% propolis and beeswax has been found to be beneficial, the propolis absorbed by the skin works as an anti-inflammatory, analgesic and the heat is said to increase joint mobility by improving blood circulation in the area affected.

Dosage to help:
Daily up to 2 grams of propolis capsules or tablets.

Alzheimer's

It was reported as far back in March 1998 of an extraordinary event with propolis given to an elderly patient by Sister Carole of the Little Sisters of the Poor to alleviate a recurring chest infection which was not responding to antibiotics. Within days the chest problem was resolved, but the propolis treatment triggered a positive side effect on the patient who had symptoms of Alzheimer's. She appeared more alert and had a more of an interest in her surroundings and other patients.
Sister Carole continued to give propolis to a further twelve patients at St.Josephs Home in Newcastle, England, and ten more patients in Lambeth London all suffering from the same condition. All showed a marked improvement to their quality of life. The improvement in the patients condition was gradual and positive.
"I'm not claiming to have found a magic cure, but the results have been extraordinary", says Sister Carole. Don't you love stories with a happy ending?

Asthma

If you do not have an allergy to honey or bee stings then Asthma could be treated effectively with propolis by inhibiting the inflammatory process present in respiratory ailments.
Since taking propolis, an Asthma sufferer for many years felt as though he had 'new lungs'.

Dosage to Help:
Daily up to 2 grams daily. Tincture of propolis is a more concentrated form and can have a more immediate effect to stave the onset of an asthma attack.
Many people take 500 mg per day. I take double this dose, simply to stay well and keep my immune system in trim.
Authorities recommend a break every 6 or 8 weeks for a week at a time.

Bronchitis

Honeycomb cappings which contain raw honey and pollen (a higher antibacterial value than pasteurized - none heated - honey which lacks important enzymes) and propolis inhalations was used to treat patients with this condition in Russia. The group was split up 56/48. The former were treated conventionally, the latter with the cappings.

Those taking the honey and propolis inhalations were cured up to 4 days earlier than those treated conventionally with fewer relapses.
Dosage to Help:
In the absence of honeycomb cappings, an alternative could be Manuka honey, produced by bees pollinating the Manuka tree in New Zealand. According to research and the latest studies at Waikato University Research Unit by Professor Molan, are showing that this honey with a UMF® value (Unique Manuka Factor) with a minimum standard of 10 gives an increased antiseptic and antibacterial properties, stimulating the body's immune system and helping the body to deal with infection.

Cancer

As previously mentioned, cancer in beekeepers can be rare. A survey of thousands of beekeeping societies in Germany found that 1 in 3,000 reported having cancer, as opposed to the US where 1 in 4 persons will have cancer in their lifetime. This could be for a variety of reasons. The use of their own pure honey cappings which contains propolis, pollen, and even exposure to sting venom may have something to do with beekeepers resistance to cancer.
It has also been reported that treatment with a high factor Manuka honey be taken on an empty stomach and 3 gram capsules daily can ease the cancer treatment.

Chronic Fatigue Syndrome (ME)

An ME (Myalgic Encephalomyelitis) survey, sent privately to James Fearnley of Beevital, published the results of 58 of their members in 1997. All Aged between 26 and 67, and having been diagnosed with ME for between 11 months and 14 years.
Of the participants 12 were bedridden or housebound whist nearly one third were very poorly.
They took between 1-12 grams of propolis per day in tablet, tinctures and tablet form.
Out of the 58, 53 reported that taking propolis had made an improvement to their condition almost immediately; one reported an adverse effect and 4 patients were not aware of any change.
Out of 22 people who said that they had reduced or stopped their treatment, 18 reported deterioration, with an immediate improvement once they had restarted treatment.
The effective suggested dosage by the authors was about 3000 mg per day, but the more seriously affected patients found relief at between 8-12 g per day.

Patients reported greater mobility, an increase in energy, and a reduction in infections.

Coughs and Colds

A propolis spray has been found to be affective also; propolis and lemon soothers (lozenges) are now available. A persistent cough can be helped by gargling with a propolis tincture mixture 4 or 5 drops taken diluted in a glass of warm water.
The best results can be obtained by taking 1 to 2 grams of propolis per day.

Cuts

A non alcoholic tincture can be applied this will sting less, because of is antibacterial properties it will reduce the risk of infection and effect quicker healing.

Cystitis

Urinary tract infection, an inflammation of the bladder, usually affects women, but can affect either sex or age groups. It is usually treated with antibiotics. Taking two 2000gram capsules daily has been found to be a good alternative, and then one capsule a day long term dosage as a prophylactic (to keep the symptom at bay)

Dental Treatments

The use of propolis in dentistry has become the most popular areas of clinical research in the world and has been the traditional treatment for hundreds of years.

More recently, a German researcher Dr.Schmidt in 1980 conducted a double blind clinical trial of a propolis mouth rinse. The study showed patients with gingivitis (gum inflammation) improved significantly with this method of treatment. Three years later Romanian researchers confirmed the trials of Dr.Schmidt, with propolis and royal jelly.

In 1990 a Russian study with propolis confirmed it's potency in root canal fillings because of the anesthetic effect and bone generating properties.

Another study in 1991 carried out in Japan on rats found that those given a propolis/water solution, showed less dental deterioration than untreated rats.

Now, up to the minute studies in the UK, have been carried out effectively, thanks to the work by Dr.Philip Wander.
The patients of Dr.Philip Wander who runs several dental practices in the Manchester area of the UK can thank their lucky stars that he has become a worldwide authority in the use of propolis for a wide range of dental problems.

Dr.Wander, amongst his many qualifications gained his Diploma from the Faculty of Homeopathy in 1994 in London England, specialises in natural dental techniques that minimise discomfort and improve oral health. He advocates the use of propolis mouthwash or gargle for temporary relief of sore throats and gums and halitosis (bad breath).

As long ago as 1995 he reports the experiences of a growing number of his colleagues who are using propolis and tinctures to treat painful oral ulcerations, dental trauma and root canal therapy.

He states that propolis has a slight anaesthetic effect as tinctures can be applied to ulcerated areas with a cotton wool bud where other preparations are not so effective at staying in place. Treatment can then be continued by the patient at home.

Another application where he has achieved success is in treating gum inflammation of erupting wisdom teeth. The beauty of this treatment is that pain is relief is immediate much to the relief of grateful patients.

His 'paper' in January 2005 "Health from the Hive, Applications of Propolis in Dentistry" highlights the growing problem of tongue and lip ulcers aggravated by body piercing. His photographs in this article illustrate the before and after effect of tincture application which provides a physical resin barrier and showed significant healing three days later.

His other much publicised paper "Taking the Sting out of Dentistry" (very apt!) mentions other dental applications of propolis tincture such as accelerated healing of extraction sockets, denture stomatitis (inflammation of the gums which can form under dentures...thrush), mouth ulcers, cold sores, and treating dental decay, particularly in children's teeth.

Dr.Wander is the only dental surgeon to have received a fellowship in Dental Homeopathy FFHom from the Faculty of Homeopathy in London.

He has written numerous articles promoting dental homeopathy and holistic dentistry, and **now** advises other practitioners on a consultancy basis.

Eczema

Propolis cream can have an amazing effect on dry Eczema. Just apply daily together with up to 2 grams daily capsules at the start, for a few days.

The Daily Mirror in their Health Extra column reported on the case of their 2 year old with chronic Eczema. "His skin was red raw and we hadn't had a proper night's sleep for two years" said his father. "But were amazed at the results when we bought a jar of propolis – we could see the difference the next morning".

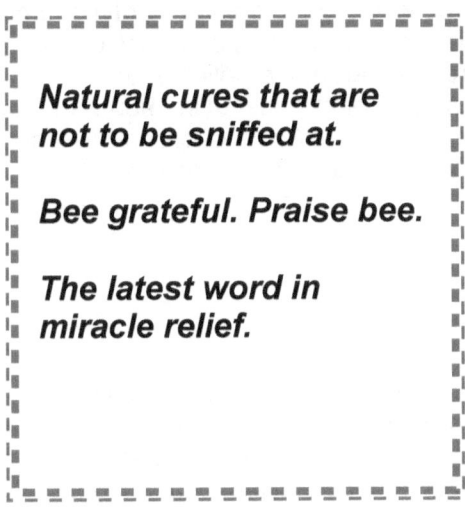

Natural cures that are not to be sniffed at.

Bee grateful. Praise bee.

The latest word in miracle relief.

Endometriosis

(A tissue similar to the lining of the uterus which is found elsewhere in the body causing infertility, painful periods and pelvic pain)
A paper presented to the 59th annual meeting of the American Society of Reproductive Medicine in 2003, by Dr. F.M. Ali of the Ain Shams University in Egypt, researched the results of 40 female patients for more than 2 years. These patients were given 500mg. of propolis twice daily or a placebo for six months.
The study showed that among those given the propolis, 60% became pregnant as opposed to 20% given the placebo.
There were no side effects recorded and the trial concluded that bee propolis could be an effective treatment for infertility and mild endometriosis.

Halitosis (Bad Breath)

Dr. Maximillian Kern, Ljubljana Clinic in Yugoslavia treated halitosis with propolis. Their symptoms entirely disappeared within a few days. After 8 weeks he checked all the patients again and found no reoccurrence of the problem. Regular brushing with propolis toothpaste can help the condition.

Hay Fever

Sufferers have reported a reduction in their symptoms after taking propolis, but it can largely depend on the allergy to a particular type of pollen.
Some people have found relief by taking a spoonful of local honey or local bee pollen a month or so before the start of the pollen season.
Dr Remy Chauvin treated a number of patients in 1980 with a propolis extract for seven days, eight doses daily of 250 mgs of propolis extract. The patients symptoms were completely alleviated in most patients.
Dosage to Help:
As above in capsule form.

Laryngitis

The treatment of sore throats, tonsillitis and acute laryngitis has found favor with the use of propolis. Positive effects have been very noticeable
Researchers in Rumania in 1975 treated over 200 patients with propolis. Ten percent of each group was treated by conventional methods. Those treated with propolis recovered more quickly than the control group.

Dosage to Help
Gargle with a solution of propolis tincture in warm water. The solution can be swallowed for added effect.
Throat lozenges are commercially available, and can be used on a daily basis as a booster.

Prostate Problems

Many men after a certain age notice that urinating and flow deteriorates. When it does start it is weak and spasmodic
These symptoms are caused by benign prostatic hyperplasia (BPH), the herbal extract saw palmetto is quite often recommended, particularly in Germany.

However propolis had been clinically tried in 1997 in Bulgaria by Mladenov on 55 patients aged between 55 and 95. All had been recommended for conventional surgery.

Honey, propolis, bee pollen and royal jelly were given to patients as individual needs were assessed. After treatment 95 per cent of patients over a period of 8 weeks no longer complained of pain and their prostates returned to normal size.

Shingles

Treatment with propolis has proved effective for this annoying complaint in both capsule form and propolis cream. Two gram capsule taken daily and the cream has the effect of eradicating the itching.

Toothache:

Using tincture of propolis on a cotton bud or similar in region of the aching tooth area. This can reduce the pain because of the anaesthetic effect of propolis until dental treatment can be affected.

Ulcers

Dr. Franz K. Feiks at the public hospital in Klostereuberg in Austria was one of the first to use propolis to treat stomach ulcers in 1978.

In a clinical study involving 294 patients he found that 90 per cent of 108 patients given a 5 percent extract of propolis 3 times daily were free of symptoms and pain after 2 weeks, compared with only 55 per cent of those conventionally treated. Dr. Feiks found that 70 percent obtained some relief in 3 days.

I have mentioned Manuka honey from New Zealand previously in this book. A high UMF® (Unique Manuka Factor) value is recommended for oral use, the greater this value the more effective the treatment. This product is usually available from good health food stores.

Warts

Warts are benign growths of the skin caused by a virus and can cause pain and discomfort if not treated.

Dosage to help:

A topical application of propolis, at least 50% tincture in alcohol solution applied twice a day for two weeks has proved to be effective.

Wounds

The ancient Egyptians and Greeks over 4000 years ago recognized the healing properties of raw honey applied to burns and wounds, boils and slow healing sores and abscesses.

When the healing processes of modern antibiotics have stopped working the medical profession has turned to honey products.

Contrary to popular belief, one of the best ways to heal a wound is to keep it moist. Now, dressings are available which are made from a highly absorbent seaweed material saturated in a high grade Manuka honey from New Zealand which the experts say kills bacteria and speeds up the healing process.

Clinical trials show that Comvita Medihoney™ eradicates MRSA from venous ulcers.

Treatment to help:

Also tincture of propolis should be used owing to its antibacterial properties, and to reduce the risk of infection.

Propolis is now known to inhibit to inhibit the growth of MRSA which as we all know is a serious problem in hospitals. Maybe it will become the answer to this common infection!

Chapter 9

Your Questions and Answers

FAQ about Propolis

Dosage.
As propolis is classed as a food supplement and not a medicine there will not be dosage instruction on the packaging.
I have indicated the dosage for the ailments that I have listed both from my own experience and those of others.
The allergy specialist Dr. McEwen the allergy specialist, recommends a minimum dose of 1500 milligrams i.e.1.5 grams. But Russian doctors who we know have decades more experience with the use of propolis are known to prescribe up to 9-10 grams per day for some serious conditions.

In my experience, I have found it beneficial to take up to 3grams per day for 2 weeks before a long flight, or when flu is prevalent and then taper down to my normal dose of 1 gram per day in capsule form, with no ill affects.

Allergies and Propolis?

As we now know propolis is a natural food from the hive, and like all foods there is a possibility that a small number of people could have an allergic reaction to it, but toxicity is rare. It has been estimated that 1 person in 2,000 can have a reaction to propolis and bee products, including beekeepers themselves. An allergic response can manifest by skin inflammation, redness and itchiness
In fact a paper was published in 1967 by the Department of Dermatology in Edinburgh following up on the allergic reactions developed by beekeepers found that rashes were only prevalent during seasonal times when handling honeycombs and bees. Similar cases and patch tests were carried out by the same Department which confirmed the allergies. In most cases during the winter months (when not attending the hives) the condition was not evident.

Is it Safe for Children?

It is recommended NOT to give propolis to children, until they have blown out their first candle! and then in a small dose to test for allergic response. In Murat's paper propolis the Eternal Natural Healer he recommends half the adult dose however taken, and then build it up gradually.

Is Propolis available for Vegetarians?

Capsules and tablets are available for vegetarians. Propolis liquids are recommended for a more immediate effective response, i.e. in the case of an asthma attack or severe infections.

Is Organic propolis available?

Not readily available. As bees forage over an area of twelve square miles or so, it is not possible to guarantee that the bees forage within a completely organic environment which has to be free from all herbicides and pesticides.

Is it safe for animals?

Much of the research on the use of propolis on animals has been carried out in Europe, Eastern Europe and China with some notable results, particularly in the treatment of cattle, pigs, poultry and sheep.
Many veterinarians are turning to natural products to treat our animals,
pets including birds, cats, dogs, fish, rabbits and guinea pigs.
performance animals, racehorses, riding horses, and racehounds.
In particular, farm animals, including cattle, pigs, sheep, and poultry.
Problems with antibiotics are again driving this movement.

Veterinary practitioners are concerned both about the decreasing effectiveness of antibiotics as well as the public concern of antibiotics in food, particularly, how they may be increasing our very own resistance to antibiotics.

Reports on the treatment of farm animals and pets have been reported with some considerable success, particularly useful in cattle production and treating skin disorders, infections and wounds.
James Fearnley's book "Bee Propolis" Natural Healing from the Hive, gives more detail for those wishing further information.

Is raw propolis available?

Raw propolis chips can be obtained from your local bee keeper. Just check first to make sure that it is clean and comes from an area which is environmentally friendly. Your local Beekeepers Association could help you here on both counts. The taste is not unpleasant, and when chewed has a slight numbing/ anaesthetic effect on the mouth. After a short time it changes to a consistency not unlike chewing gum.
This method of taking propolis is ideal for combating sore throats, gum disease, mouth ulcers, and even bad breath (halitosis)

Propolis preparations.

Propolis tinctures are the easiest to make and most common preparation and it has the maximum therapeutic effect.
Propolis chips broken into small pieces and store in the freezer for a few days until it becomes brittle. Use a pestle and mortar to grind the chips or a coffee grinder can be used.
The most commonly used solvent is alcohol. Food grade alcohol **must** be used, **not denatured alcohol** as this contains dangerous chemicals to prevent it being consumed.
Use about 40 grams of propolis powder and mix it with 100 ml. of 70 per cent proof alcohol or higher proof, and leave it in a warm dark place for 7 to 14 days stirring daily. Use as little heat as possible as this can tend to damage its potency. Be aware that alcohol is highly inflammable so keep away from a direct flame source. For home use you can use vodka or gin as the solvent suspension.
After two weeks the solution can be filtered though fine muslin or coffee filters can be used. Store the solution in a dark brown bottle in the fridge for a few days, and then filter again using as fine a filter as possible.
Store the liquid in the bottle away from direct sunlight. In this way it can be stored indefinitely.
Take a few drops daily to keep coughs and colds at bay usually in a warm drink, or you can use it in your own honey to improve the potency of the product.
The tincture can of course be applied to cuts and grazes infections and wounds.

Water Extract------ Rather than use alcohol, water can be used. Using alcohol externally as suggested above can sting slightly on open wounds, so propolis Sprays with water may be more conducive using this method.

Method.. Use 10 to 15grams of propolis powder mixed with pure filtered water, after 24 hours, and shaking regularly, filter the solution as above.
The solution can be mixed with a small amount !:20, mint, eucalyptus, lavender etc, to be used as a nasal spray.
Use a mechanical spray to treat burns and skin infections.

General Advice.

The best way to take propolis is to try it gradually, only small amounts for the first few days. Afterwards, slowly increase the dosage assuming there were no side effects.

Chapter 10

Conclusion

Conclusion

Serious problems of bacterial resistance have been revealed in all our hospitals worldwide for the past decade, MRSA being just one case that is being well publicized.

We face a worrying crisis of overuse and total dependence on chemical medicine, but to our credit we are all becoming aware of the benefits of natural products for combating diseases.

We have seen that propolis has proved that it can alleviate many health problems with little or no side effect, and importantly it does not kill friendly bacteria unlike antibiotics.

Propolis is not a cure all solution to our ailments. A magic bullet does not exist, but propolis could play an important role in the future, both in the home and in our hospitals and has vast potential for human health.

I sincerely hope that my research has proved helpful in making you aware of a natural food supplement which could alleviate possible health problems now, and in the future.

PROPOLIS is truly God's gift to us all. Bee Well and remain in good health.

Chapter 11

Selected References

SELECTED REFERENCES

Dr. Ali F.M. Ain Shams University of Egypt Treatment of Infertility and mild endometriosis. October 2003.

Dr. Remy Chauvin 1980. Subject Propolis in the treatment of hay fever. Apiacta. 15/101/3

Osmanagic Izet 1976. Report on Influenza and its preventative properties Sarajevo.

Dr. Maximillian Kern, Ljubljana Clinic in Yugoslavia. Treatment of halitosis with propolis

Dr. Philip Wander 2005. 'Health from the Hive'. The applications of propolis in Dentistry.

Dr. Leonard McEwan 1996. The Allergy specialist. London. Treatments with propolis at his clinic.

James Fearnley 2001 'Bee Propolis' Natural Healing from the Hive by Souvenir Press.

Dr. Bernard Jenson PhD. 1994. In his book 'Bee Well Bee Wise. Meeting with Russian beekeepers and their remarkable lifespan.

Dr. Philip Wander 1995. Paper. 'Taking the Sting out of Dentistry'

Murat, F. 1982. The uses of propolis. Propolis, 'The Eternal Natural Healer'.

Grange. J.M.and Davey, R.W. 1990. Journal of the Royal Society of Medicine. Positive results treating MRSA strains.

Hill R. 1977 'Propolis 'The Natural Antibiotic'. Thorsons Publishers Wellingborough England.

Choice Books and Resources

Bee Propolis. Natural Healing from the Hive. (2001) by James Fearnley. Souvenir Press.

Propolis the Natural Antibiotic (1977) by Ray Hill. Thorsons Publishers Ltd

Propolis Plus by Carlton Wade (1996) Wade & Keats Publishing Inc.

Users Guide to Propolis. Royal Jelly Honey and Bee Pollen by C.Leigh Broadhurst (2005) Basic Health Publications.

Bee Well Bee Wise (1994) by Bernard Jensen Ph.D. Publisher, Bernard Jenson.

Health and Healing with Bee Products (2002) by C Leigh Broadhurst, Alive Books.

A World Without Bees (2008) by Alison Benjamin and Brian McCallum, published by Guardian Books. A brilliant read 5* rating from me.

Association Addresses

American Apitherapy Society Inc.
www.apitherapy.org

British Beekeeping Association
www.bbka.org.uk

International Federation of Beekeepers Association
www.ibra.org.uk

Beekeeping Database
www.beedata.com

Magazine of American Beekeeping
www.beeculture.com

Apimondia, International Federation of Beekeepers Association
www.apimondia.org

Propolis Producing Companies

Natures Laboratory Ltd. (UK)
www.herbalapothecaryuk.com
www.beevitalpropolis.com

Comvita Ltd. (Bay of Plenty, New Zealand)
www.comvita.com
Stores in most major countries

The Propolis People (South Africa)
www.thepropolispeople.co.za

CC Pollen Co (Phoenix, Arizona)
www.ccpollen.com

Beehive Botanicals (Hayward, Wisconsin)
www.beehivebotanicals.com

Australian By Nature Pty Ltd (NSW)
www.australianbynature.com/au

Colony Collapse Disorder

Over the past few years the global bee population has suffered a catastrophic decline. The bee pandemic known as Colony Collapse Disease (CCD) or Mary Celeste Syndrome has virtually erased 50% or more of the bee population.

Honey is in short supply as bee workers desert their queens, and once thriving bee farms are seriously at risk.

Early in October 2006 in Crawford County, Larry Curtis lost more than 80% of his 1,200 bee colonies in six weeks. By mid November he had lost 1,000 hives and 100.000 lbs of honey.

One of Pennsylvania's biggest commercial beekeepers Dave Hackenberg of Union County, Lewisburg, found that suddenly in mid November he lost 50% of the 2,700 colonies he owns. His commercial enterprise pollinates summer blueberries in Maine, and oranges in Florida.

The pollination industry in the USA was once a $45 billion industry, but no more. Some say the bees are tired of being shunted from State to State to pollinate the Californian almond crop and fruit farms in Florida.
Some say the Varroa mite is the culprit, other pesticides, others mobile phones, GM crops, who knows.

Bees are the lifeblood of the universe and now beekeepers worldwide are demanding their respective Governments for adequate funds to solve the bee pandemic.
There have been demonstrations in Spain and France to draw attention for the need of funds to research CCD and other bee parasites.
Even as recently as November 5th 2008, thousands of British beekeepers demonstrated in front of No.10 Downing Street, each carrying their hive smokers and placards demanding more action to fix the honeybee problem.
As a direct result of this activity, the UK Government has allocated £10 million to research our pollinators including the bees.

The problem is not a new event. Bees have been disappearing since the first known event in the USA in 1869. Long before GM crops were introduced and before pesticides were used. In the UK in the early 1900's 90% of the bee population in the Isle of Wight UK were mysteriously wiped out.

But let's face it, we have been exploiting bees since the evolution of time, stealing their honey, desecrating our planet and killing them off without thought or favor. Let us respect them, and nurture their habitats.

"If the bee disappeared off the surface of the globe then man would only have four years of life left" Albert Einstein

So, this is not a new problem and I hope that the bees with our help can find their own solution.

NOTES

NOTES

NOTES